The Secret

N A T R O N

aka Sodium Bicarbonate

aka Baking Soda

Possible applications in acute and chronic ailments

Marcelo Jesus Alegre

Note

The information in this book was researched from publicly accessible sources. It concerns, above all, Natron (aka Sodium Bicarbonate or Baking Soda), which is used by scores of people for healthcare purposes. All information is provided without guarantee. The information in this book does not replace a doctor or an alternative practitioner. The author shall not be liable for damages arising from the possible applications of the measures described in this book.

**One, who places his trust in a doctor,
need not be surprised by the high costs.**

(Of course, that goes for other professions as well!)

Foreword

Renal pain, breathlessness, asthma, migraine, ailments resembling sleep apnea at night, difficulties in concentration, severe back pain, dizziness, nausea, cold hands and feet and constipation or congestion. These were my symptoms, which seemed to appear out of nowhere and threw me off the tracks quite abruptly. The many physicians, whom I met as a result, were unanimous: Psychological problems! But, I was of a different opinion...

Doctor: "I do not find anything. You probably have a psychological disorder. To me, it looks like a posttraumatic disorder." Me: "I don't think so. In that case, wouldn't I have other symptoms, such as sleep disorder or nightmares or so?"

Cardiologist: "Your pulse is quite high, 120 per minute. And it's steady. Are you anxious?" Me: "Me? No! Why?" He: "It's a clear symptom." Me: "Do I look like I am anxious? Am I trembling, sweating or do I look restless in some way?" He: "No, but my diagnosis is clear." Me: "Are there other possibilities?" He: "Yes, there are many, but in your case, it's anxiety."

In the consultation during the prescribed 24-hour ECG, the Senior Cardiologist grasped the incorrect analysis – thus, that of another patient(!) – and declared: "Quite clearly, an anxiety disorder!" Me: "Excuse me, but pick up the paper, which has my name on it." She grasped another diagram: "As I said before: Psychological problems." Me: "What does the curve show with regard to the sleeping time?" She: "Slept through seven hours." Me: "Do you think that a person afflicted with anxiety can sleep through seven hours? Where does the anxiety go at night?" She, angrily: "Accept the fact, finally! Do something about it."

Further visits to various medical specialists always yielded the same results. To all of them, my ailments or symptoms seemed to be triggered by my anxiety. Eventually, I referred myself to a psychiatrist. And then I felt a bit queasy.

Psychiatrist: "At the moment, I do not see what could be triggering your ailments or symptoms. Here, just take these (tantalized me with pack of neuroleptics)." Me: "I probably do not need them." He: "Is your psychological strain not severe enough?" Me: "It has to be something else." (Ok, that's probably what most people say...)

Moreover, my queasiness led me to old friends, to a spiritual healer and an alternative practitioner. In meditative and hypnosis sessions, both of them found no evidence of an anxiety disorder.

"There is clearly something wrong", I said to myself. "There has to be something else that needs to be clarified and/or discovered". The question to myself was: "What else?" Thus, in this case, what could still be worth considering with regard to these ailments/symptoms, other than psychological problems? Over and over again, I posed this question to myself - and to the others -.

Finally, after months of search, I stumbled upon a concept, which seemed to explain the ailments/symptoms to the full extent and which the professionals did not even know or perhaps did not wish to reveal. This concept was called the acid-base-balance. I had never heard of it before. It is just not possible to know everything.

Thus, the unnoticeable hyperacidity of many years – the latent acidosis or even tissue acidosis (acidosis = hyperacidity in technical terminology) – could have caused my ailments, which led to the acute hyperacidity (acute acidosis). Following this, for days and nights, I searched the books, scientific journals and the internet for further information. And I concluded:

The doctrine of the acid-base-balance is part of the professional secrecy of many specialists in the healthcare and pharmaceutical industry. Or they do not know it themselves.

And then it happened, that the word Natron flashed on my radar. Each and every application of Natron that I discovered was almost unbelievable. Consistently amazed, I have now compiled in this book every application that is propounded in the area of health. Moreover, I found it fascinating that not a single person I had spoken to about Natron and the hyperacidity of the body even knew of the effect – and many of them did not have a clue that it even exists – of this remedy and of hyperacidity. Needless to say, Natron is not a miracle cure. Nevertheless, it is not possible to simply dismiss its positive effect on the "acidic" body and on an unhealthy lifestyle.

Already for a hundred years, it has been known that the hyperacidity of our organisms can result in health impairments, which can manifest in many forms. A book[1], which I have found, dates back to the year 1933! An important reason for this hyperacidity can be found in our lifestyle: We eat too much and, at the same time, we have unfavourable food items, such as sweets and spaghetti on our plates, and coffee and alcohol in our cups and glasses. There is good literature available on the topic of hyperacidity, and one can find excellent websites concerning this subject on the internet as well. If you are interested, you will see how diverse and ingenious are the dietary advices, and what else you can do to benefit yourself. If you are hearing it for the first time, I have briefly discussed in the annex the issue of hyperacidity and what can be done to combat it. Likewise, in the annex, I have dwelt upon the highly diverse and hidden reasons, which could severely disrupt the acid-base concept of our body.

The content of this book shall not be deemed to be an advice to ingest and/or use Natron, and one should also not get the impression that all the problems can be solved by using Natron. In fact, it should open up your mind. Stay critical and search for solutions. At times, there are ways

---

[1] A friend in need, Facts worth knowing about ARM&HAMMER baking soda as a proved medicinal agent, 1933, https://fb.docs.com/PFAM

to get out of a situation, which come to light only after tedious and lengthy search operations.

Please pay particular attention:

There are many possible uses of Natron for your health. A major point of criticism in the use of Natron is that the absorption of vitamins and minerals can be impaired. Natron itself is low in nutrients. That is why, a separate intake of various micronutrients, if necessary, has become a part of your daily ritual. Moreover, if medicines have been prescribed to you by your doctor, then discuss with your doctor, pharmacist or alternative practitioner whether you can take Natron.

Natron should not be taken during pregnancy or lactation period. The same applies to people suffering from high blood pressure. Similarly, Natron is not suitable for children up to the age of five (other sources even state up to the age of 12). However, even here, it applies to the individual case. Do not hesitate to tell your doctor about the effects and treatment potential, if you think that it could help. As for the rest, Natron is not suitable for long-term use. As soon as the acute symptoms subside, a break is recommended. In most cases, it happens after around two to three weeks.

Furthermore, - according to my research - Natron changes the pH-value in the digestive tract, as well as in the kidneys. This could disrupt the absorption of the active ingredient, as well as the excretion of some substances. (Acetylsalicylic acid, mineralocorticoids, diuretics, alpha-sympathomimetics, anticholinergics, tri- and tetracyclic antidepressants, barbiturates, ciprofloxacin, captopril and quinidine, glucocorticoids, H2-receptor blockers).

In any case, discuss the administration of Natron with a doctor or an alternative practitioner, if you are suffering from any health disorders and are taking medications for that purpose.

Diarrhea, flatulence, abdominal pains and nausea are mentioned as the rare side effects. Perhaps, in this case, the dose was too high.

Further worth mentioning[2]:

- Do not drink Natron more than six times in 24 hours. If you are over 60, three applications are considered to be the upper limit.

- Do not take Natron for more than two week (predominantly applies to higher dosages).

- Natron can lower the level of your vitamins and mineral nutrients, B vitamins and chromium are mentioned in particular.

- Do not take Natron, if you have to eat a diet that is low in sodium (in case of high blood pressure). In case of long-term use, the sodium level would increase and the calcium level would decrease.

- Persons who are suffering from edema, liver diseases and/or renal diseases should not ingest Natron.

- Drink Natron only when it has completely dissolved in the water.

- Take Natron only on an empty stomach; one hour before a meal and three hours after a meal.

- High doses of Natron may cause diarrhea. If this happens to be the case, reduce the dosage by half or take a short break.

- Consult your doctor, if you experience swelling on the feet, weakness, labored breathing or nausea.

The author assumes no liability for the applications of Natron, which are described in this book. In case of doubt or if you have any further

---

[2] World Wide Web, diverse sources

questions, inform your doctor, pharmacist or the alternative practitioner about your intentions.

Table of Contents

What is Natron

Natron was omnipresent even in the times of our grandmothers. This white powder was available in pretty much every household. This was mainly because of the enormous variety of its possible applications and also due to its extremely low price. Natron was used as a cleansing and disinfecting agent, as well as for personal hygiene, odor neutralization and for cooking and baking, to name just a few examples.

Nowadays, unfortunately, Natron has been sidelined. Kind of exactly like the unsurpassable recipes of our grandmothers. Therefore, it is not surprising that we have to really discover it once again. The Internet mainly provides us with the household tips and tricks. However, its medical *possibilities* should not be underestimated. Above all, it fights against the hyperacidity of our body and lifts the acidic environment towards the healthy alkaline state, which can restore our youthful buoyancy - at least, to some extent -.

Natron is also known as the baking soda, whereby, it is important to mention that the common backing soda contains other substances as well. Therefore, only use pure "baking soda" called Natron or Sodium Bicarbonate.

In Switzerland, Natron is sold as powder, which can be purchased at a very low price in the drugstores, pharmacies and major supermarkets. In the neighboring countries, it is also available as Kaiser-Natron or Bullrichsalz, either as a powder or even in tablet form, with or without mineral supplements.

The foodstuff industry has codified Natron as a food additive **E500**.

What can Natron do

Natron is fully equipped to balance the ph-value of our body. In other words, it has an alkaline effect. An excess of acid can (in most cases, after decades of latent, minimal excess of acid) lead to a diverse range of diseases, including osteoporosis, arthritis, asthma, up to tumor diseases, such as cancer, which thrives particularly well in the acidic environment. Regular administration of Natron shifts the pH-value towards neutrality and enables our body to lift its fitness to an unimaginable level.

In order to understand the effect of baking soda, first of all, one must be aware of the consequences of a highly acidic body. A constant acidic pH-value leads to the congestion of spleen, liver, heart and kidneys. In order to buffer these acids, the body deprives the bones and tissues of the urgently needed minerals, and directs them to another urgently needed location in the body. Thus, in a manner of speaking, the minerals move around in circles because no other minerals are directly available. This primarily involves calcium, magnesium, sodium and potassium. This "redeployment" of endogenous substances can lead to chronic diseases, such as osteoporosis, kidney stones, loss of muscle mass and impairment of muscular functions, as well as heart diseases, diabetes, cancer, arthritis and other diseases.

Where does Natron come from?

Natron is a naturally occurring salt deposit. On the American and African continents, such deposits are found in nature and are mined together with other products. In Europe, Natron is produced in other manners. It is produced from common salt by replacing the inherent chloride with carbonate. Unfortunately, my knowledge of chemistry is not sufficient for a better explanation.

Who needs Natron?

Natron can be used by almost every human being because, in general, we are all acidotic - unless you are already very particular about your lifestyle. This book deals with the health-related benefits of Natron. Most people might think that they do not need it because they are fit as a fiddle. That very well may be the case. Nevertheless, in a considerable number of people, especially in the industrialized nations, the latent hyperacidity is a concern, which should not be underestimated. In the annex of this book, you will find a list of medical conditions (doctors and health insurance companies also refer to them as diseases), which, in many cases, can be attributed to this latent, thus invisible and creeping hyperacidity.

What does "I am acidotic" actually mean?

The acid-base balance of our body is briefly presented in the annex. There are many books written on this subject. As a layman, I cannot provide an in-depth report on this topic. This area is rather knowledge-intensive. Moreover, there are slight divergences with regard to what is good and what's not, but those are just details.

We are talking about the acids in our body, when substances are capable of making us sick. Studies suggest that approximately 8 to 10 persons in our society are mildly to severely acidotic, thus they have already been toxified. Harsh as it may sounds, but it hits the nail on the head .

A major part of our acid load is a direct result of our dietary habits. Much of what we enjoy, builds up acid during digestion in the alimentary tract, the so-called acid residue. What's more, there are medications, which very often have an adverse effect on the acid-base balance. Obviously, the medications work, but one should keep that at the back of one's mind. Stress, anger, rage, grief, sugar, coffee, cigarette smoke, cola drinks and car exhaust and so much more make us "acidic". And then there is hydrogen. When we eat acidic food (actually, it should be called foodstuff, which contains acids), we add hydrogen ions to our body. These then adversely affect the excretory system organs (intestines, liver, kidneys, lungs and even the skin). Many medical conditions, which we know by different names, could be a consequence of the above. Depending on the constitution of a person and his habits, the harmful substances are excreted optimally or even sub-optimally from the body. You will find a list of such diseases in the annex.

The hyperacidity can also lead to a mineral deficiency and/or even a deficiency of base-forming minerals in our organism.

In addition, the flow properties (viscosity) of the blood and/or of the red blood cells changes. A persistent hyperacidity causes the miniscule red blood cells to become sluggish, until they are no longer willing to act flexibly. These elastic erythrocytes, as the red blood cells are called in the technical jargon, are unable to flow smoothly through even the tiniest of blood vessels (capillaries). Among experts, it is then understood as the acidotic rigidity of erythrocytes.

If you are about the same age as I am, just visualize the Dutch family of shapeshifters Barbapapa, who could change into any shape they please and slip through the minutest of holes.

As an example of this rigidity, I will mention the loss of hearing: In the inner ear, this capillary is extremely thin. Normally, where the red blood cells were just able to flow through, this poses an ever-increasing obstacle now, until, finally, it is not longer possible. This is the physical cause of the hearing loss. The persons affected are acutely acidotic and the immediate visit to the doctor is inevitable.

Medical science distinguishes between two types of acidosis. It speaks of respiratory or metabolic acidosis, whereby the respiratory and metabolic acidosis can be acute and **measurably** disturb the pH-value. The latent acidosis still does not get detected by all the medical professionals because it is undetectable in the blood. It is not objectively diagnosable using scientific methods. This means that no diagnosis can be made. The possible diagnoses are, namely, clearly classified.

Latent acidosis

The latent acidosis – in other words – means the tissue acidosis. Thereby the acids and the toxic substances are gradually and unnoticeably shifted into the connective tissue and stored there, until they can be excreted. This happens, for instance, in case of a fasting or any other form of dieting, even, for instance, in case of a flu or a fever or when we sweat. Then, this form of hyperacidity affects almost all of us. Problems in excreting these acids, under certain circumstances, may result in minor to severe health-related problems, which then cannot be attributed to any apparent cause. As already mentioned in the case of hearing loss, this tissue acidosis can occur locally. Lumbago, back pain or swollen joints should be mentioned here as an example for many other manifestations.

The medical science does not seem to have recorded this symptomatology in the study books. Moreover, as a layman, I ask whether this latent acidosis could lead to one of the two below-mentioned medically acknowledged acidosis.

Respiratory acidosis

The respiratory acidosis can occur due to the poor breathing habits or due to impaired pulmonary functions (asthma, medications etc). If, for any reason whatsoever, a person is no longer able to breathe abdominally on a regular basis, that is to say, has shallow breath or breathes too rapidly, he will develop problems with his wellbeing sooner or even earlier. This form of acidosis can occur due to persistent thoracic breathing. In addition, sleep apnea is a cause of this form of acute and measurable acidosis.

Metabolic acidosis

This acute metabolic acidosis is manifested by the kidneys being unable to cope with the metabolization of the acids, either because they have functional problems or because far too many acidic products have to be metabolized at once. In such cases, it also affects those persons who constantly perform extreme feats of strength or endurance. The respiratory, as well as the metabolic acidosis can be detected in the blood by a decrease in ph-value. In medical science, this form is treated by using the sodium bicarbonate, in other words Natron.

What must be observed

In the following chapters, I will present some areas of application of Natron for your health and your wellbeing. My researches resulted in a plethora of applications. Natron can be used a remedy for the acute treatment, as well as for preventive healthcare. Let yourself be surprised by the numerous possibilities offered by this powder!

But:

Natron does not replace a healthy lifestyle and, above all, any well-balanced and the majority of alkaline diets!

The use of Natron is primarily advised as a short-term remedy, either in case of acute ailments or even as a temporary treatment. Long-term intake is not recommended due to mineral deficiencies. But I have also come across usage tips, which make it possible to take Natron on a daily basis and/or apply it externally. But let me repeat: It is better to lead a healthy lifestyle than to deceive the body, by constantly feeding it "Natron", into believing that it is healthy, which it is not in fact.

It may be worthwhile, by all means, to experiment with Natron. As a start of deacidification and as a cure, two or three times a year, - in my opinion - Natron can hold its ground without any problem.

Herxheimer reaction - Initial worsening of the symptoms

When, as a result of appropriate remedies, bacteria, fungi or parasites die inside the body, the toxic substances, with which we are already contaminated, could cause various ailments. In this process, quite frequently, not only these organisms are attacked and eliminated, but even the heavy metals accumulated in the body (especially existing in the fungi). The reaction can be clearly manifested and can afflict the person affected much more severely than the already existing symptoms of the disease. This is referred to as the initial worsening of the symptoms. As this term already implies, it concerns a temporary deterioration of the health. For instance, in case of a heavy metal contamination, theses accumulations now detach with the fungi, and pass through the intestines towards the exit. Under certain conditions - if they are not similar to a diarrhea-like situation -, parts of these heavy metals are transported into the bloodstream. Furthermore, the liver, the urinary tract and the colon are excessively afflicted. As a result, the body looks for other organs, which can support during the process of detoxification. These are lungs, skin and paranasal sinuses (Aha! In case, you are wondering now, why you are constantly suffering from cold.)

There are a number of indications of the initial worsening of the symptoms, such as, for example, headache, diarrhea, fever, itchiness, joint pains, nausea, night sweats and many more.

How to maintain control over the Natron intake

You can keep an eye on the acid-base balance of your body by keeping a check on your urine. For this purpose, there are the so-called indicator papers, also referred to as the pH-value test strips. Depending on the acid-base status (precipitated hydrogen ions), these paper strips change their color. You can buy them in drug stores and pharmacies. A measured pH-value of 6.8 or less is considered to be acidic, and a consumption of alkaline supplements, such as Natron that is mentioned in this book, is advisable. **A value of 7.5 – 8.0 once a day is desirable[3].** At the beginning of the measurements, it is ideal to determine the value during every visit to the toilet, thus you will see how your ph-values vary during the day.

It helps to create a table. The more acidic the value, the higher the daily dosage. In an ideal case, you would not need Natron. But you must also bear in mind that the nature and quantity of the foodstuff and fluids, stress and dietary supplements also directly influence the ph-value.

The measurement of our saliva would be another option. However, the environment of saliva is completely different, or rather a different pH-value. In this book, I shall confine myself to the value contained in the urine. Although this is not comprehensively convincing. Basically, it only states how much hydrogen is excreted. A lower pH-value is equally acidic. This is what relates to the so-called extracellular deacidification, that is to say outside the cells. In this theory of explanation, the intracellular acid load is also explained for this purpose: The acid within the somatic cells. These would have to be achieved using potassium and magnesium[4].

---

[3] Jungbrunnen Entsäuerung: Wohlbefinden rundum durch ein harmonisches Säure-Basen-Verhältnis [Deacidification, a Fountain of Youth: Overall Wellness through a Harmonic Acid–Base Balance],
Kurt Tepperwein, 2001
[4] Dr. Jacobs Weg des genussvollen Verzichts, Dr. med. Ludwig Manfred Jacob, 2013

How to test whether I am acidotic?

There is a test, with which you can easily detect whether you are hyperacidic. For this purpose, mix one teaspoon of Natron in a glass of water (2 dl) and drink it immediately. The taste will take time getting used to. Rinsing with a plain glass of water will bring the facial expressions back on track. If the value measured in your urine is not at or exceeds beyond 7.5 wihtin an hour, then in the circle of alternative practitioners, you are considered to be hyperacidic and a treatment seems to be inevitable in view of this fact. The corrective remediation takes time, therefore, bear the following in mind:

What you have done to your body over decades cannot be made to disappear within just a few weeks or months!

Natron in case of acute and chronic ailments

Heart attack

The heart attack is a consequence of hyperacidity[5]. The heart attack is aggravated by stress, whereby stress means different things to different people. However, in reality, in a vast majority of cases, the primary cause of the heart attack can be found in the unfavorable dietary habits, which leads to the much mentioned hyperacidity. In case of hyperacidity, the red blood cells, as already mentioned, lose their elasticity (viscosity), and, finally, can no longer squeeze through the blood vessels. It results in congestion.

As an immediate measure, the ingestion of a fast-acting agent, Natron, appears to be sensible. The advice in this regard:

Prompt consumption of 1 teaspoon Natron, dissolved in ½ a glass of water. If the person affected is no longer able to drink it on his/her own, then the solution should be dripped into the corner of that person's mouth.

Stroke

Just as the cardiac infarction, a cerebral infarction is supposed to be a consequence of an acid flooding, which the body is no longer capable of processing[6]. The red blood cells, which begin to coagulate in case of chronic hyperacidity, no longer penetrate the vascular walls resulting in congestion in such a case.

---

[5] Jungbrunnen Entsäuerung: Wohlbefinden rundum durch ein harmonisches Säure-Basen-Verhältnis [Deacidification, a Fountain of Youth: Overall Wellness through a Harmonic Acid–Base Balance],
Kurt Tepperwein, 2001
[6] Jungbrunnen Entsäuerung: Wohlbefinden rundum durch ein harmonisches Säure-Basen-Verhältnis [Deacidification, a Fountain of Youth: Overall Wellness through a Harmonic Acid–Base Balance],
Kurt Tepperwein, 2001

The immediate measure is same as described in case of a heart attack: 1 teaspoon Natron, dissolved in ½ a glass of water, drink if possible, otherwise administer into the corner of the mouth using a small spoon.

Hearing loss

A loss of hearing can arise as a consequence of, among other things, stress, noise or an infection. A localized hyperacidity in the inner ear is considered to be responsible for this ailment. In the event of acute problems, immediately consult your doctor. However, before doing that, you could drink the Natron solution, 1 teaspoon in a glass of water, as well as soak a piece of cotton wool in that solution and insert it in the ear affected[7].

During my search related to the hearing loss, I have read that a low-pitched or a high-pitched whistling sound, which, in most of the cases, is equally indicated in both ears, can be manifested by an exposure to heavy metals. In this context, one might think of mercury in the dental amalgam fillings, as well as lead and cadmium in the automobile exhaust emissions. Heavy metals could be treated, among other things, by ingesting algae, for example, AFA-Algae or the chlorella pyreneidosa

Migraine

As soon as the first signs of migraine are detected, mix one teaspoon of Natron in a cup of warm water. Drink it immediately, followed by a glass of water.

Biliary colic

In case of biliary colics, which are accompanied by vomiting, one can provide relief by dissolving one teaspoon of Natron in 4 dl of warm water (never above 60°C / 140°F), and drinks it in several small sips.

---

[7] Jungbrunnen Entsäuerung: Wohlbefinden rundum durch ein harmonisches Säure-Basen-Verhältnis [Deacidification, a Fountain of Youth: Overall Wellness through a Harmonic Acid–Base Balance],
Kurt Tepperwein, 2001

I have come across the fact that in many cases, a gross vitamin C deficiency could be responsible for the formation of gallstones. Therefore, it is advised to take vitamin C daily. Ideally, if required, take a stomach-friendly supplement. Of course, the best option is to block the path of the acids!

Kidney function

According to an article, a <u>university</u> found out that the intake of Natron could strengthen and/or support the kidney functions[8]. Therefore, the dialysis patients would have to be hospitalized less often for the in-patient treatment. The article dates back to the year 2009. According to the above, a daily dose of Natron should improve the renal function. Yet another <u>report</u>[9] related to the same study.

Gout

Gout flare-ups and pains could be alleviated, if you mix 1/4 liter of water with 1/2 a teaspoon of Natron and drink it right away. Depending on the severity of the ailments, repeat up to four times a day. Take an extended Natron bath every now and then.

If the kidneys are overworked in the excretion of the uric acid, as in case of other ailments as well, it can lead to gout. Gout is considered to be a protective and warning mechanism of the body. Due to a constant excess of acid, crystalline structures are formed (uric acid crystals), which lead to inflammation near the joints and are extremely painful.

Burnout

The burnout is a classic case related to the excess of acid in the modern times. The science does not present any definitive diagnosis, when it is said: You are burned out! Furthermore, the doctors, pharmaceutical giants or even health insurance funds never refer to this mechanism. Since, as in case of other symptoms, the excess of acid points in the

---

[8] http://www.qmul.ac.uk/media/news/items/smd/17693.html
[9] http://www.dailymail.co.uk/health/article-1200287/Daily-dose-baking-soda-stop-kidney-patients-needing-dialysis.html

direction of unspecified and even threatening acute symptoms, these symptoms are now recognized as an individual disease. Thereby, in most cases, the burnout is nothing other than the result of a longstanding hyperacidity, which (apparently) presents itself with an acute symptomatology. Nevertheless, even specific events in the life of a person could induce a burnout.

As soon as the first signs of a burnout are detected (there is a wide range of them), immediately take one teaspoon of Natron and mix it in a large glass of lukewarm water.

This solution is intended only for the immediate alleviation of the symptoms. Take remedial measures to counter the hyperacidity of your body.

Radioactive contamination and soil contamination

In case of radioactive contamination and/or in case of elevated radiation, Natron should be an effective remedy to protect yourself from the hazardous contamination. In general, the kidneys are the first organs to experience the damages after a radiation poisoning caused by uranium. Natron has the ability to bind the uranium and to support the kidneys in their excretory work. Therefore, if your live near a nuclear power station: Be sure to stock up on Natron. As an additional measure, magnesium baths also have a supporting effect[10].

In case of strong radiation exposure, full baths with Natron should be taken. For this purpose, pour approx. 400 - 500 g (14 – 17 oz) Natron in the bathtub. Take four to five baths per week and (only) in case of really elevated radiation. Under normal circumstances, these dosages are quite high.

The issue of radioactivity is a delicate subject, and I suppose the authorities can deal with the truth generously. We only need to think of the Fukushima or Chernobyl meltdown. Quite certainly, the radioactivity was carried hundreds and thousands of kilometers (miles) away. Perhaps

---

[10] http://www.radiation-antidote.com/anti-radiation-baths.html

even much further. How can we measure this as a layperson? Not everyone has a dosimeter at home.

Much more inconspicuous are the uranium enriched agricultural lands, which are inconspicuously emanating these radiations. Would you have thought that? The agricultural lands are fertilized with uranium-enriched phosphorus fertilizers! Although, hopefully, there is still a long way to go, until the carrots start to glow, but I am afraid that we will observe the effects on our bodies at a much earlier stage. The Swiss farmers have already been fertilizing their farmlands using phosphate fertilizers for decades. Two to five tons of phosphate fertilizers are used annually. The manure leaches into the groundwater and, eventually, reaches the lakes and tap water as well. Especially with regard to Lake Thun in Switzerland, people have been wondering for ages now why the whitefish has been exhibiting atrophies and are developing mutations. Perhaps that could well be a possible reason.

The phosphate fertilizers are derived from North Africa and Russia. Measurements taken in Switzerland showed that the values of this material were ten times above the normal values. The report is available on the website of the Swiss Federal Office for Agriculture [Bundesamt für Landwirtschaft]: Human and environmental impact of uranium derived from mineral phosphate fertilizers[11]

Incidentally, the Swiss military is "optimally equipped" to face a nuclear impact: Every soldier receives an emergency ration, comprising of chocolate (that is obvious in any case) and cookies. And these cookies really pack a punch. They are, in fact, Natron cookies. A former Head of the Swiss Military Department was even of the opinion: "We have the strongest army in the world!" No wonder, having the knowledge of such a secret tip.

---

[11] https://www.admin.ch/gov/de/start/dokumentation/studien.survey-id-623.html

Flu

In case of flu, Natron helps quite quickly. If you are experiencing aching muscles and limbs, reaching for this white powder is worthwhile. But this miraculous white powder can be taken even to prevent the flu.

If you would like to, just try the following in case of flu:

Day 1: Take half a teaspoon of Natron dissolved in a glass of water, six times a day, at an interval of 2 hours distributed over the course of the day. (Thus, half a teaspoon every two hours.)

Day 2: Repeat the same, once again!

Day 3: Reduce the dosage: Take half a teaspoon in the morning an half a teaspoon in the evening.

From the 4th day - If the flu has not yet subsided -, take half a teaspoon of Natron only in the morning until the symptoms have gone away.

Note with regard to flu[12] [13]

Since the beginning of the 20th century, there has been some evidence that the flu can manifest itself only in the presence of a certain degree of acidosis. Perhaps this explains why there are human beings who have never come down with flu. In this study, it is also mentioned that persons, who took Natron on a regular basis, did not show any symptoms of flu, even when flu was "raging" all around them. It makes it seem as if the flu virus does not stand a chance in case of human beings having an intact acid-base balance.

Hay fever

As soon as you detect the first signs of hay fever, take one teaspoon of Natron in a glass of warm water on an empty stomach, and drink another glass of water immediately afterwards[14]. You should do this every day,

---

[12] Arm & Hammer - Baking Soda Medical Uses, Dr. Volney S. Cheney, 1924
[13] http://www.bibliotecapleyades.net/archivos_pdf/commoncold_volney.pdf
[14] Durch Entsäuerung zu seelischer und körperlicher Gesundheit, Dr. med. dent.

until the allergy season is over. Do not take even a day off because the symptoms will return immediately. However, bear in mind that you should not follow through with it for more than two to three weeks. However, I know people who take Natron for an extended period of time.

Tip:

Take a balanced base powder every day. In recent years, there are many different products available in the market. You can take the base mixture every day on a long-term basis. This will help your physical environment to stay within a healthy range and provide you with the most essential minerals. If you stick to that, you should have no more complaints next year, as far as the hay fever is concerned.

Allergic asthma

In case of allergic asthma[15], the same theory applies as in case of hay fever because this form of asthma evolved from decades of hay fever condition. However, a complete recovery can take several years. As a rule of thumb, it is reckoned (for the complete deacidification):

Your body requires 10% of your lifespan for the complete healing, provided that you are leading a healthy lifestyle.

Allergic asthma is considered to be based on the increased histamine production due to the chronically acidified organism. Thereby, the bronchial tubes cramp up. In case of non-allergic asthma, the attack is supposed to be caused by the acid load itself.

Beck/Ingeborg Oetinger, 2014, 22.Auflage
[15] Jungbrunnen Entsäuerung: Wohlbefinden rundum durch ein harmonisches Säure-Basen-Verhältnis,
Kurt Tepperwein, 2001

Note by the layman writing this book: Possibly, in case of a suspected diagnosis, the histamine intolerance might be reviewed as well. Histamine intolerance is - not entirely unfounded - a subject of highly controversial discussion.

Bronchitis

Natron can also be inhaled[16]. In case you are suffering from Bronchitis, then nebulize a solution containing Natron. Inhaled Natron is supposed to have a mucolytic and relieving effect. For this purpose, there is a so-called "Alternativ-Inhalator" (German name). Search for this term on the internet and you will find the suppliers of this excellent device. Perhaps you also have knowledge of other inhalers and nebulizers.

Here is the recipe for the solution: 2 teaspoons of Natron, dissolved in half a cup of water. For the alternative inhaler: Add a few drops in the inhaler and start inhaling.

Snoring

Drink one leveled teaspoon of Natron dissolved in 2 dl of water. Immediately thereafter, "chase" it with another glass of water. It can help in reducing the snoring, if it is triggered by the degradation of the acids. Administer this solution approx. two hours after dinner or before going to bed. Based on my own testing, I have found the first suggestion to be better. But as is well-known, proof of the pudding is in the eating.

Note: Measure the pH-value of your urine when you wake up. If it is greater than 7.5, then reduce the quantity of Natron in the evening. Even this application is recommended as a regimen and not as a permanent solution.

sleep apnea under suspicion

In case of sleep apnea, the educated opinions are divided. It seems clear that the specific cause has still not been found. However, the connection

---

16

http://healyourselfathome.com/HOW/THERAPIES/SODIUM_BICARBONATE/sodium_bicarbonate_nebulizing.aspx with the respiratory acidosis is supposed to be clear. The author is of the opinion that the latent acidosis can definitely lead to sleep apnea. Even in this case, Natron could bring relief in the first phase. From my own personal experience, I would suggest that the daily breathing exercises (above all, the abdominal breathing), as well as exercises to strengthen the jaw, neck and tongue muscles can achieve excellent results. On Youtube, there are some really cool videos[17] [18]for this purpose.

These risk factors are considered to be certain[19]:

- Overweight, large neck circumference
- Narrow nasopharyngeal airway space (for example, due to enlarged tonsils)
- Persons who drink excessive alcohol, especially in the evenings
- Persons who regularly smoke
- Sleeping pills or sedatives
- Relatives with sleep apnea syndrome
- Male version of the human kind

On closer inspection, one could imagine that, in such a case, the hyperacidity may have already started to take effect deep down a long time ago. A detoxification/deacidification and heavy metals detoxification is necessary!

Altitude sickness

If you are suffering from acute altitude sickness, drink water treated with Natron. This will help in alleviating your symptoms. Take 1/8 teaspoon in a liter of water. Drink one glass of this solution upon manifestation of the first signs.

---

[17] https://www.youtube.com/watch?v=g42ooYpPF7Q
[18] https://www.youtube.com/watch?v=zlJyslYGbLc
[19] http://www.lungenliga.ch/de/krankheiten-ihre-folgen/schlafapnoe/ursachen.html

Premenstrual syndrome (PMS)

The menstrual problems experienced by women every month, which could become unbearable for them, could, in the opinion of the author, be mitigated by taking Natron.

Thus, if it is unbearable: Try to help your body in the elimination of the acids (menstrual bleeding) by taking one teaspoon of Natron in 5 dl of lukewarm water. This should be the usual procedure on the first manifestation. However, one should bear in mind that the acid producing foods should be eliminated. By doing so, you stand a good chance in bringing this miserable PMS to its knees.

You will find more information on this mechanism of menstrual bleeding in the annex.

Cellulite

The insiders have known it for a long time: Cellulite is often a consequence of unfavorable dietary habits. It is quite certain that the dimpling, predominantly in the female skin, is induced by acid. The skin is essentially an important excretory organ for the substances, which the body does not want to have. Now these substances accumulate subcutaneously and wait until they are eliminated, such as, for instance, by means of sweating.

If cellulite poses a stress for you, then let Natron work for you.

Regular full baths with Natron (approx. twice a week) could actually work wonders! Mix 100 g (3,5 oz) of Natron in the bathtub and pretty soon you will look years younger and, most probably, feel young as well. This, of course, applies to all genders.

Psoriasis

According to a British study, Natron is also effective against Psoriasis[20]. The itchiness and skin irritations were alleviated by regular full baths. For that purpose, mix half a cup of Natron in approx. 37°C warm bating water.

---

[20] http://www.ncbi.nlm.nih.gov/pubmed/15897164

Tonsillitis

As a household remedy, Natron is also effective in case of tonsillitis. Bacteria and fungi do not like Natron at all. The acids in the throat and nasopharyngeal area are neutralized, which can lead to an alleviation of tonsillitis.

Dissolve one teaspoon of Natron in a glass of lukewarm water and gargle for approx. 30 seconds, and then spit it out. Repeat this a few times. Gargle this solution several times a day.

Muscle soreness

Directly after the physical exertion, it helps if you dissolve one teaspoon of Natron in a glass of water and drink it immediately. Thus, the muscle soreness would be outsmarted, which is, in fact, the consequence of a hyperacidity of the muscles.

Alternatively, a full Natron bath is a reasonable option to counteract the muscle soreness. Stay as long as possible in the bathtub. But it should be, at least, one good hour.

Insect bites

Painful bee stings can be relieved immediately, if you mix Natron with cold water into a viscous paste and apply it directly on the bite.

Why do mosquitoes bite some people more than the others and some not at all? To a significant extent, this is due to body odors released via human sweat. The mosquitoes – as well as other species of insects – are attracted by the odor of human beings. Firstly, we emit CO_2 by breathing. If the mosquito has flown towards this emission, our body odor plays a key role, if it smells of hyperacidity (acetone, lactic acid or butyric acid), then the mosquito just swoops in to attack. From now on, you will no longer be surprised by the afflicted human beings, who are covered in mosquito bites. You now know an important factor: Hyperacidity! Even ticks could develop a ravenous appetite when they smell these odors. A further observation of the author relates to the head lice. Since not all of our children were afflicted with these cohabitants, rather only one out of four, I am of the opinion that the abovementioned body odors emitted by sweat could bring the lice into frenzy. Interestingly, exactly this child was covered in mosquito bites as well.

Minor burns

Minor burns, like the one's I get from the oven every now and then, could likewise be treated by a viscous Natron paste. Just apply this paste on the affected area and leave it to dry out. This will prevent blistering. Add two teaspoons of Natron in a glass of water, stir it and pour it on the affected area.

Alternative, mix one teaspoon of Natron with one teaspoon of vegetable fat, spread it over the affected area, and leave it to work for approx. 10 minutes. The pain goes away and there are no blisters either.

Sunburn

If you were out in the sun for a long time, then you can do the following: Dip your t-shirt in a Natron solution and wear it. This will alleviate your pain.

Another, somewhat more convenient method: Mix 4 teaspoons of Natron in a cup of water and spread it over the affected areas.

Heartburn

Stir just a little more than a leveled teaspoon of Natron in a glass of warm water and drink it in one go. As an alternative, you can also drink the Natron mixed water in sips.

Eczema

A full Natron bath can be helpful in case of eczemas. For this purpose, you will need 100 g (3,5 oz) of Natron to mix in the bathing water. No further additives are required.

Fungal infections on the skin

A full Natron bath is recommended, twice a week. Bathe in it for at least one good hour. Afterwards, just rest in bed. Another effect of a full bath is that with regular application, your skin will look youthful and fresh. Who does not want that?

Fungal infections of the gastrointestinal tract, thrush / for example, Candida Albicans

Should you be infected by Candida Albicans or any related fungi, then a high dosage of Natron may be an expedient remedy. I myself have successfully tested the method of "Trojan horse". However, these fungi are insidious and could develop time and time again, if you are not terribly careful with them. Thereby, the diet plays a key role.

For the purpose of Trojan horse, you will need one teaspoon of Natron, which you have to mix in 3 teaspoons of maple syrup. Take one to a maximum of three teaspoons of this mixture, spread throughout the day. Use it for a maximum of two weeks. In the second week, just take one teaspoon of this mixture every day.

Athlete's foot

Natron is effective against a variety of fungal infections. As a preventive care, you can sprinkle Natron powder in your shoes. Thereby, a pinch of this powder in the socks will also do no harm.

If the athlete's foot itches between your toes, just mix Natron into a paste: 1 full teaspoon of Natron and ½ a teaspoon of water. Rub this paste between your toes, let it dry and wash it after 15 minutes. Do not forget to dry your feet thoroughly before slipping them into the shoes again.

One more variant:

Powder your feet with Natron, rub and/or massage it gently into the skin and leave it to work for approximately a quarter of an hour. Afterwards, wash your feet thoroughly. Do it twice a day.

Alcohol hangover

If you were unable to quit it yet again. Then Natron can put you back on the track: Add one teaspoon of Natron in a glass of water and add a dash of lemon juice to it. Drink it quickly! (You know how it's done)

Cancer, tumor diseases

An article by the National Center for Biotechnology Information[21] reported that the formation of metastases could be inhibited and/or reduced. On the internet, you will find reports, according to which some types of cancer were made to disappear with the use of Natron. It may not have been confirmed scientifically, however, there could be a grain of truth in it.

There is an Italian Oncologist[22], who expressed the suspicion that Candida Albicans aids and abets in the growth of tumors. The fungus is, so to say, a preliminary stage to cancer. This doctor goes even further: According to him, the tumor could even be the original fungus itself.

It can be inferred from another article[23] that there is a clinic, which also integrates Natron in the treatment: "At the clinic, we use 12 g of pure Natron mixed in 2 cups water, along with a low-cal sweetener of your choice (because it tastes quite salty). Sip this mixture over the course of an hour or two and repeat for a total of three times a day."

Since cancer is supposed to develop in an acidic environment, the intake of Natron is considered to be a preventive measure!

You will further find an interesting report here[24] on the topic of pH-values, growth of tumors and treatment possibilities with Natron and other substances. It is also mentioned that the way to combat a tumor is to keep the ph-value measured in the urine above the value of 8 for quite some time. This value should be kept constant at this level for five days[25].

---

[21] http://www.ncbi.nlm.nih.gov/pubmed/19276390

[22] http://www.canceractive.com/cancer-active-page-link.aspx?n=2719

[23] http://www.drwhitaker.com/7-baking-soda-health-benefits/

[24] http://www.health-science-spirit.com/de.krebstherapie.htm

Cigarette, alcohol and drug withdrawal

Because of the diversity of possibilities, which I have stumbled upon within the course of my researches, it is definitely conceivable for me that a course of treatment with a high dosage of Natron can make a withdrawal somewhat more bearable, without having to resort to substitutes.

An experiment to make the cigarette smokers give up smoking, which was conducted already in 1979, demonstrated unambiguous results. After three weeks, almost all the smokers, who were treated with Natron, gave up this vice, whereas both the other comparison groups were still actively smoking. In this study, the experts expressed the suspicion that a high acid load in the body could be related to an increased urge to smoke. However, to a large extent, the success of this study was based on the fact that all the subjects were prepared for the imminent withdrawal by means of psychotherapeutic preparatory measures for approximately two to three weeks. Nevertheless: With the help of Natron, it felt a lot better[26].

Even though I am not a medical expert, I get a creeping suspicion that the use of Natron could enable similar treatment opportunities for alcoholics and drug addicts.

Be that as it may be: In order to quit smoking or even just to see for a moment, how many fewer cigarettes do you need, dissolve one teaspoon of Natron in 2.5 dl of water and drink it twice a day between meals.

Flatulence

In case of gaseous symptoms, try the following: Mix half a teaspoon of Natron in a glass of water, and add juice of one squeezed lemon. Then pretty soon, windlessness will prevail. Hopefully, this is not the calm before the storm.

---

[25] http://www.blissful-wisdom.com/ph-8-level-cancer-cure-with-sodium-bicarbonate--baking-soda.html
[26] http://www.spiegel.de/spiegel/print/d-40350634.html

Constipation / diarrhea

Constipations can be alleviated, if you add half a teaspoon of Natron in a glass of water and drink in one go. Strangely enough, this same procedure also shows the loose motions who the master really is. In such a case, hyperacidity has two faces. Constipation and diarrhea are even possible in alternation.

Chickenpox

Is your child suffering from chickenpox? Then prepare a Natron bath for him/her.

Inflammation of the throat, difficulty in swallowing

If you are facing difficulties in swallowing, take a glass of warm water mixed with one teaspoon of Natron and gargle with it every three to four hours.

Canker sores

Dissolve one teaspoon of Natron in a glass of warm water. Gargle with it vigorously. You can do this several times a day. This will heal the canker sores much faster.

Pimples

Prepare a creamy paste using Natron. To make it, add one teaspoon of Natron in approx. 3 teaspoons of cold water. Apply this paste on the pimples, briefly massage it in and let this mixture work for some time. Applying it for half an hour twice a week would not be bad. You may apply a moisturizer after the Natron treatment[27].

Common cold, nasal congestion

Mix one teaspoon of Natron in a glass of warm water and pull it through the nasal cavity, it will loosen the thick mucus. Subsequently, bend forward with the head facing down and blow the mucus out. Do this several times, until the glass is empty.

---

[27] http://de.wikihow.com/Pickel-mit-Natron-bek%C3%A4mpfen

Cystitis / inflammation of the bladder

Bacteria love a slightly acidic environment. This seems to the major reason why so many people complain of cystitis or inflammation of the bladder. The environment in the bladder [cyst] is the perfect breeding ground for the bacteria.

You can very effectively alleviate the symptoms of cystitis by mixing Natron in water and drinking it daily until the infection has disappeared.

The recommended dosages may vary. If you like, start with half a teaspoon of Natron dissolved in one cup of water. You can also dissolve a full teaspoon in one cup and drink it.

Halitosis and caries

In case bacteria in your mouth are responsible for a foul smell, then rinsing your mouth with Natron may help you. By the way, Natron is also effective against the smell of onions and garlic.

Mix one teaspoon of Natron in one cup of non-carbonated water and gargle with it a few times.

This also reduces the risk of caries.

Natural deodorant

Natron drives away foul odors! A person who knows the scene well uses it by mixing one teaspoon of Natron in water, until it turns into a kind of crème, which he then, for instance, rubs under his armpits or on his feet.

Protect your tooth enamel / Natron toothpaste / White teeth

Some foodstuffs, such as, for example, lemon juice, temper with your tooth enamel. In order to protect you tooth enamel, mix baking soda in water and gargle it several times a day.

Alternatively, you can brush your teeth using Natron toothpaste and, in doing so, it may do some good to your tooth enamel as well.

By using Natron, you can also make your teeth whiter:

Fill two-thirds of a cup with Natron and slowly add water to it, mix it until it forms a matter resembling a toothpaste. If the taste does not work out right away, do not worry. Because here again, someone knew what to do. Add approximately 10 drops of peppermint oil to this paste. Then briefly rub it on your teeth, leave it for five minutes, and then rinse it thoroughly. This application is recommended once a week.

Natron for the preservation and maintenance of health

Full bath

For a full bath, add approximately 100 grams of Natron powder to the bathtub. This will refresh and rejuvenate your skin and complexion. This bath has a detoxifying effect on your entire body. Just remain in the bathtub for, at least, one hour with a temperature of approx. 37°C (98,6 °F). The longer you bathe in it, the better it will be! Pretty much two such rejuvenating baths per week would be optimal.

Footbath

Fill a bowl with warm water. Add one teaspoon of Natron for every liter (33 oz) of water. Your feet will thank you. This is really effective against the cracks in the skin and the burning sensation in the soles of the feet. It is also effective against sweaty feet. The sweaty feet are also an indication of acid degradation, thus, if required, we have to support them in the best possible way.

Mouthwash / Gargle

Mix 1 teaspoon of Natron powder in a glass of lukewarm water, and your mouthwash is ready. Gargle several times. Daily use will prevent mouth odors, caries and inflammation in the mouth and throat area.

Nasal douche

For a nasal douche, you will require the following ingredients and paraphernalia

- 1 teaspoon sea salt
- 1 pinch of Natron
- 2 dl lukewarm, boiled water
- Plastic syringe

To perform the nasal douche, tilt your head to one side and squirt the solution into the nostril that is on top – wait for approx. 20 seconds, then tilt your head to the other side and perform the same procedure. Daily application will help in keeping your nose clear.

Alternatively, as described further above: Add one teaspoon of Natron in a glass of warm water and rinse your nose with it.

Trojan horse

For the Trojan horse, you will require one teaspoon of Natron, mix it with 3 teaspoons of maple syrup. Take one to three teaspoons of this mixture spread throughout the day. Take it for a maximum of two weeks. In the second week, just take one teaspoon of this mixture every day.

By using this little trick, the acidic, anaerobic (subsisting in the absence of oxygen) cells "pounce" upon the sugary mass and, in the doing so, come too close to the admixed Natron, which causes them to die by elevating the pH-value.

According to my researches, one can easily perform this Trojan horse once or twice a year as a preventive measure. Over an extended period of time, it pushes the pH-value to 7. 5 upto 8.0 on the acid-base balance scale. As a result, other undesired bacteria, fungi and other pathogens are either driven away or destroyed.

The Trojan horse apparently also severely impacts the tumor. A tumor – also referred to as the cancerous growth – develops as a result of uncontrolled cell growth, a proliferation. There is (at least) one doctor, who claims that cancer is actually a fungus, which multiplies at an incredibly accelerated pace. Its favorite food is sugar. It consumes much more sugar as compared to the healthy cells. (In this context, simple carbohydrates are mentioned, which immediately convert into sugar in the body.)

An American study conducted in the year 2009[28] with regard to the effects of orally ingested Natron on the breast and prostate cancer states

---

[28] http://www.curenaturalicancro.com/pdf/bicarbonate-increases-tumor-ph-and-inhibits-metastases.pdf

that the formation of metastases was able to be inhibited and the pH-value of the tumor was increased. Another study from the year 2013 even proved that the tumors can be shrunk[29].

Add Natron to your drinking water

In the USA, there is an "insider's tip": Take one liter (33 oz) of non-carbonated drinking water(!), add just a pinch of Natron to it and drink this water by noon.

Enema

Natron is equally well suited as an enema to balance the pH-value. Take two tablespoons of Natron and dissolve it completely in two liters (67 oz) of warm water. To learn how to perform an enema at home, you can ask a specialist, buy a book or surf the Internet. The enema kit does not cost much.

Another interesting practice that I have stumbled upon is as follows: Rotate (while lying down with the enema) along the longitudinal axis by 90° every 10 minutes. It should be effective against tumors in this area, and thus reaches all possible corners.

Children's laughter

Especially beneficial for your health is a child's laughter. To induce this contagious health measure, you need a 1.5 L PET bottle, vinegar and Natron.

Fill up the PET bottle with a finger's breadth of vinegar, add 5 teaspoons of Natron and put a balloon over the opening of the bottle. The mixture produces carbon dioxide and fills up the balloon. You will become a hero and the children will never forget it!

---

[29] http://cancerres.aacrjournals.org/content/early/2013/01/01/0008-5472.CAN-12-2796.abstract

Contraindications

A responsible use of remedies, in this case, use of Natron, always weighs the risk of therapies vis-à-vis the risks of existing alternatives, as well as vis-à-vis the risks of refraining from a therapy. A complicated sentence, which, however, has earned its place at this point.

If you have any concerns, then ask someone who should know better. Thus, in such a case, visit a doctor or an alternative practitioner who you trust.

The contraindications and specific characteristics can be found in the introductory chapter.

Annex

The concept of the acid-base balance of our body

Hyperacidity of our body

A large number of chronic courses of a disease originate in an acidic environment and, in fact, acute manifestations, such as, for example, lumbago(!) are in reality clear symptoms of long-term hyperacidity. The intake of minerals is important after and even during the deacidification of the body. On the one hand, this happens by adapting a diet and, on the other hand, the hyperacidity, which has been existing for decades now, requires a supply of minerals because a balance no longer appears to be sufficient only through diet. Dietary supplements are very useful resources in such a case. In such a case, consulting an alternative practitioner or a nutritionist is probably the best solution for most of the affected persons.

Hyperacidity is a symptom

Already the hyperacidity itself is symptom and emerges as an individual medical condition in action, such as, for example, gout or constipation. It has many manifestations. In such a case, it is imperative to identify and eliminate the causes of hyperacidity.

Causes of hyperacidity

The reasons of hyperacidity are often not apparent at the first or a second glance, perhaps not even at a third glance. The medical and pharmaceutical scene is cleverly using this fact to their benefit by demonstrating a symptom-oriented thinking, intending to treat these symptoms and even developing the pills for that purpose right away. This is probably very well justified and helps the person affected in many cases. But only when the person affected really tackles the actual causes of his ailments, a sustained improvement can be achieved.

Anxiety

Nowadays, the production of anxiety is cultivated in pure culture, and, in fact, in all the spheres of life. In the mass media, we read about war, conflict and accidents of all kinds. It seems almost as if the human race is just ill-fated. We have to be afraid of losing the job, of economizing and of becoming impoverished. We are afraid of getting our computer infected by a virus, of getting robbed. Would you believe the things we are afraid of! You see:

Fear rules the world (and your physical functions)!

Who does not know this? Nevertheless, fears are part of our lives, we continue to evolve with each fear, which we overcome.

Stress

Quite a number of scientific and non-scientific papers have already been written on stress. It is not worthwhile to write more about this topic in this book. What stresses us - and what does not - depends not least on our thoughts, emotions and situations, in which we find ourselves.

Breathing

When fear and stress exist, the breathing rhythm derails eventually. The breath becomes shallow and the breathing rate becomes more rapid. The air is no longer drawn into the abdominal region, rather turns around from the thoracic region. A lot of things happen during the process: The exchange of oxygen and carbon dioxide is impaired, the degradation of acids is prevented. By breathing correctly, even the undesirable substances are neutralized.

Diet

The diet has already been mentioned above. Do not forget: Every human being has different needs. Needless to say, this also applies to the kind of diet. Some get it, some don't.

Too much or too little exercise

Hyperacidity of the body is very common, in particularly, in the performance sport. This almost cannot be counteracted through diet alone. Of course, professional athletes have an advantage here. That is to say, they can rely on the specialized knowledge of the support staff. But many amateur sportspersons are unable to process the acids - in this case, among others, the lactic acid - on a long-term basis. At some point, the organism becomes weak. Often precisely in competition, for which one has strenuously prepared for a long time, the entire capacity is required.

Even too little exercise can lead to hyperacidity. Therefore, if you are an enthusiastic couch potato, go for a walk nevertheless. In such a case, walking would be a fairly optimal solution.

Acid-Base equalizer

I am quite sure you know about the stereo system equalizers. As a music listener you determine the treble and bass of the tone of your favorite music. This is, more or less, how a slide controller acts for your well-being. Let us assume, the different slide controllers control the values of anxiety, stress, breathing, diet and exercise. Each adjustment of one of these levers influences the functions inside you. If you slide the controller No. 3, you would have to probably reposition one or the other controller optimally. And just as the settings of the preferred tone, even the adjustment for your body is really an arduous task under certain circumstances. However, if it is perfectly tuned, you will develop an unimaginable power!

The problem is, as already mentioned, that every "adjustment of a controller" can force the readjustment of the other controllers. In addition, the fact remains that not every human being functions in the same manner and/or not every individual needs the same adjustments. Maybe the nature has deliberately configured it in such a manner. While one person needs to party till he/she drops, the other has numerous opportunities to get away from it all.

Pay attention to your own equalizer and find your personal settings. Although it is not possible to make recommendations, however, in principle, you can, when breathing, eating and exercising, apply that lever first of all, with very fine and controlled changes to the slide controller.

Diseases or symptoms of hyperacidity[30]

Allergies, asthma, hay fever, high blood pressure, cellulitis, diabetes, inflammations, joint pain, bone fractures, grey hair, skin impurities (pimples), hair loss, infections, headache, concentration problems, exhaustion, muscle cramps, migraine, menstrual problems, heart burn, sleep disorders, underweight, overweight, digestive problems, gum inflammations, pale skin, swollen or cold hands or feet, dark circles under the eyes, osteoporosis, back and joint pains, spinal disc problems, constipation, diarrhea, flatulence, gallstones, urinary stones, internal and external fungal infections, rheumatism, lumbago, mood swings, tinnitus, thrombosis, tumors and so on so forth.

This list is long and not even complete! But you see how important it is to keep an eye on the acid-base balance, to reduce the acid and to pamper the base. Please do not think that something like this cannot happen to you. Even if you do not experience any symptoms, just find out your acid-base values from time to time.

How many people go to a doctor for some diseases, and the doctor prescribes medications, and a considerable part of these medications is probably not even needed. These even include placeboes, thus the sham drugs. The medicinal and pharmaceutical industry has found names for many diseases, which are actually symptoms(!), and wants to diagnose these diseases and fight them as well. But if the hyperacidity is the root of many evils, why are then, time and again, new remedies created to fight the symptoms arising as a result of hyperacidity? You will not be surprised: A lot of money can be made with it and one can lead the people by the nose. And all that under the pretext of helping. By saying thing, I do not intend to denigrate the relevant scene in any manner whatsoever. I, too, am happy that there are medications and doctors.

---

[30] Internet, various sources

Nowadays, earning lots of money,
economic growth
and increasing your profits
is more important than anything else in the world

In the end, not everything can be attributed to an acidic body environment, but, as it seems, it plays a significant part. Especially in case of chronic ailments, which manifest themselves in the form of acute attacks like a bold out of the blue, it is worthwhile to investigate on your own.

Chronic and unnoticed hyperacidity, also referred to as the latent acidosis in the technical jargon, is the - as already mentioned - the basis of many ailments. This means permanent stress for the body.

A possible effect is the formation of undesirable fungal cultures in our digestive system. One of these fungi is Candida Albicans, a genus of yeast fungi. It gradually multiplies rather unnoticeably, till it achieves the status of uncontrolled proliferation. It can then infect all the mucous membranes. Have you, by any chance, had a stuffy or a constantly runny nose? Have you perhaps had a coating on your tongue and asked yourself, what could that be? Are you suffering from constipation or diarrhea, or even from both? Shortness of breath or asthma? This fungus further afflicts the joints. By any chance, do you know about the tennis elbow, or do you have painful thumb joints or shoulders (predominantly the left side)? The list of ailments is long. The symptoms differ from person to person. This also makes it so difficult to get the idea that the hyperacidity could be the cause of all this.

This Candida Albicans exhibits a particular characteristic. It binds heavy metals. Why this is so, I was not able to research conclusively. Probably, it is a protective mechanism of our body. In case of chronic hyperacidity, the heavy metals could no longer be transported to the exit.

Personally, the following appears probable to me: With regard to the fungus, we can extract an example from nature. The nature actually likes to plant the fungus in bodies where vast amounts of dirty or toxic substances are deposited. For example, using certain species of fungus, an oil spill can be cleaned up relatively fast and in an economically sustainable manner, or can mitigate a toxic soil contamination. In this sense, it means that the fungus can and will protect us from the toxic heavy metals, until a solution could be found for the stressful situation.

The fungus: A warning signal and a protective mechanism at the same time!

However, there is an important point in case of the regression of the fungus. If one succeeds in making the fungus beat a hasty retreat and/or remediate the environment, it also releases the super-elevated levels of heavy metals and other toxicities, which leads to additional ailments, which resemble or intensify the toxicity symptoms (Herxheimer reaction).

This fungus was already described in ayurveda, the medical science and philosophy of ancient India. Experts of ayurveda call it **AMA,** a component of digestive toxicities. The proliferation of fungus in our body seems to have been known even thousands of years ago, and was treated with meditation exercises and by making changes to dietary habits. The cause of AMA was seen as a combination of overeating, stress, mental and emotional tension, as well as anxiety.

Special circumstances affecting women

The regulation of acid-balance balance has a special significance in case of women. Once the menstruation period starts, the female organism adapts itself to bear offspring. The toxic substances, notably the acids and toxics, are isolated from the body and are eliminated once a month. A fantastic mechanism, which ensures that the body is kept free from toxic substances.

However, there is also a danger for the females here. Due to this natural plan, it can happen that during the pregnancy and after the period has ended, the female is tormented by health disorders, which are exhibited quite clearly every now and then. Quite often, these resulting symptoms are not identified as symptoms of hyperacidity. In such a case, the individual "classic symptoms" are, for example, osteoporosis caused by the resulting mineral deficiency, cellulite and weight gain due to deposits of undesirable substances, which are now no longer eliminated periodically.

Heavy metal toxicity due to hyperacidity[31]

The consequences of a heavy metal toxicity (for example, due to platinum and palladium in the catalytic convertors in our automobiles, mercury in dental fillings, lead, cadmium, arsenic in cigarette smoke or at shooting ranges and nickel in jewelry) strongly resembles the effects of hyperacidity of an organism. Quite often, problems in excreting heavy metals can occur in case of hyperacidity. In other words, if you are on track in terms of your acid-base balance, then the body has to be capable of eliminating its toxic substances to the complete extent. Symptoms of a possible heavy metal toxicity are:

Aggressiveness, allergies, general weaknesses, chronic fatigue, lack of energy, depression, resistance to antibiotics, lack of drive, anemia, asthma, blood pressure disorders, sensory disorders (such as, numbness, cold feeling, tingling sensation), inflammations of the sinus, epilepsy, fibromyalgia, joint pains, skin eczema, herpes, cardiac arrhythmia, hormonal imbalances, hearing disorders, hyperactivity in children, susceptibility to infections, headache, liver damage, memory deficit, concentration disorders, throat and stomach pains, twitching in the mouth area (corner of the mouth), neurological disorders, internal restlessness, irritability, neurodermatitis, renal damage, psychoses, fungal infections, thyroid dysfunctions, insomnia/difficulties in falling asleep, dizziness, blurred vision, severe sweating, speech problems/slurred speech, inflammation and pain in the gums, tremors, autism, dyslexia

---

[31] Internet, various sources

Body temperature and hyperacidity

We all know that our body temperature is around 37°C (98,6°F) and that it is, of course, subject to fluctuations. Thus, for instance, when we are asleep, our temperature falls to approx. 36.2°C – 36.5°C (97,16°F – 97,7°F) or maybe even lower. That seems to be the normal case and even the guild of medicine men of the western world shares this view. However, from the ayurvedic point of view, the ideal operating temperature is between 36.5°C (97,7°F), when we are in the land of dreams, and can reach the peak point of 37.3°C (99,14°F) in the afternoon or in early evening. A small, but subtle difference, in my opinion. I know a lot of people, whose body temperature never exceeds 36°C (96,8°F), and they are exactly the people who often complain about the health problems and disorders. This is not a coincidence! Too low a temperature tempers with our power station. It weakens the immune system.

Even this chronic sub-normal temperature progresses into hyperacidity. The ayurvedic dietetics even differentiates between the foods, which exert a heating or a cooling effect on the body. This is not surprising because most of what we consume, in any case, comes out of the refrigerator. This storage of foodstuff, when we eat it unheated, inevitably leads to a drop in our body temperature. For that purpose, a distinction has actually been made between the foods, which exert a heating or a cooling effect on the body. Lists of such foods can be found on the Internet. I am not an expert on this matter. Ayurvedic dieticians or even the specialists of Chinese medicine know more about it.

At this point, let me just remind you of the connection between the body temperature and hyperacidity. Because our engine - if it is unable to establish ideal temperature - exerts itself in order to function properly, it will not harm to take the thermometer, every now and then, into your own hands (or elsewhere). Furthermore, there is a possibility that the body temperature eventually tends to drop with the years of one's life. This would be easy to explain with the knowledge of hyperacidity and/or the accumulation of the toxic substances. In any case, already as a child, it became conspicuous to me, how warm it had been in the grandma's room, and nobody knew why it had to be so.

And how do I now increase the temperature? That is relatively easy to achieve. Move your body, but do not overdo it, and certainly not near a street with heavy traffic. For example, take the stairs, instead of the elevator or board the bus one stop further. As already mentioned, you can consume the temperature-increasing foods. What can be much more difficult and can take quite a long time is the detoxification or even the deacidification of your body. Regular sauna sessions, warm baths and cold-weather clothing are further supporting measures, just as the relaxation and breathing exercises.

The detoxification works much better at 37°C (98,6°F)![32]

---

[32] 37°: Das Geheimnis der idealen Körpertemperatur für optimale Gesundheit [98.6: Ideal Body Temperature as the Secret to Optimum Health], Uwe Karstädt, 2014

What you need for the deacidification (detoxification)

First of all, it is important to bring the metabolism back on its feet. For this purpose, it is recommended to include lots of green vegetables and bitter herbs in your meals on a permanent basis. Relaxation exercises, massages, breathing training, as well as light sports/exercises on a regular basis. Just do not go overboard with the physical exercise, this is not everyone's cup of tea and can further escalate the hyperacidity. Also be careful with the fruits. It is advised to eat fruits sparingly and if you want to, eat them in the morning or as a dessert to the main course. Eating a lot of fruits does not necessarily make everyone healthier.

Natron

The Trojan horse is particularly suitable as a course of treatment, once or twice every year. Or just take it as the starting point of the deacidification course. It makes sense, above all, if you are experiencing clear symptoms.

Mix 1 teaspoon of Natron with 3 teaspoons of maple syrup, and take one to three teaspoons of this mixture spread over the entire day on an empty stomach. You can take this for a few days.

In between, when I have this feeling that it will benefit me, I take Natron first thing in the morning.

Breathing exercises

The most important breathing technique actually belongs to the category called "the most natural thing in the world"; the abdominal breathing.

It is a sign of the times that most of us, more or less, are permanently under pressure. A meeting here, an appointment there, and soon we have, once again, landed in our beds later than intended and to recover from the stress of the day gone by. After just a few hours of sleep, the alarm clock goes off on time, once again, way too early. It's the same every day. In addition, you experience restless sleep and stress before you wake up!

Due to this permanent stress, the ability to leisure slips away from us, it is recognizable by our breathing, which becomes shorter and shallower, and breaks up already at the level of our thorax. This thoracic breathing leads to the situation that the carbon dioxide exchange in the lungs cannot be performed to the full extent. If this happens for a longer period, we become acidic in the long run!

For this reason, several times a day, concentrate on taking deep breaths. This should be firmly planned in the daily routine already at the outset. As time goes by, you will get used to it and you will be breathing like a child again.

Massages

In my opinion, it does not play a significant role what kind of massage you treat yourself to from now on. You will discover the most pleasant form yourself. How about a hot-stone-massage or a Thai massage? Perhaps, even a warm oil massage or an acupressure would be something for you. There are actually a variety of beneficial and relaxing massage techniques. Indulge yourself!

Relaxation exercises

It is worthwhile to learn one or more relaxation exercises and to practice them regularly. There is, for example, autogenic training, hypnosis, yoga, meditation and many more. You will already have your favorite or you will find it soon.

Fasting days

Even as far as fasting is concerned, one should not go overboard right away. There is a simple way to eliminate the extremes: Just pick a day to fast once every month (you will be surprised how easy it is) and skip the dinner once or twice a week. In this manner, you will give your body, as already mentioned, a breather and a break from digestion.

Eat Half as Much

This method does not need to be explained in detail: Eat half of what you usually eat! This gives the body the time to metabolize everything that it needs, and does not have to move anything excess into the tissue and store it as fat for the winter. At the same time, it has more time to eliminate the toxic substances.

Basic (alkaline) food

There are actually diverse opinions on what healthy food should contain and what not. Thereby, only one thing is clear: All human beings are equal; except for the fact, what is healthy for them.

You will quite certainly find out, what is good for you or, at least, what would be good for you.

In conclusion

At this place, I have a small request once again: If you have concerns or if you are not familiar with one of the fields mentioned above, pleased make use of a professional support for that purpose.

**No one is born a master,
nor a novice either.**

By maintaining the correct pH-value within your body, Natron can enhance your overall health and wellbeing. Some health problems, such as, for example, abdominal pains, kidney stones, gout, urinary tract infections or flu can be successfully treated with Natron. It can even enhance the athletic performance.

I have personally tried some of the proposed uses and, ever since my first use, Natron belong to the list of my "Must-Have's" in the household.

On this note, I wish you all the best of health and, as Dr. Spock used to say:

Live Long and Prosper!

63756583R00035